s t r e t c h

A contemporary approach with attention to detail
Book One - The Necessary Basics

Presented by The Rejuvenators

Daphne Bashford with
Joanne Boston
Deanna Empey
and Cynthia Palahniuk

PiSco

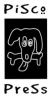

PreSs

Published by
Pisco Press
Box 130
100, 1039 - 17 Avenue S.W.
Calgary, Alberta, CANADA
T2T 0B2

First Edition

Printed in Canada

Canadian Cataloguing in Publication Data
Main entry under - Stretch
Contents: Book One - The Necessary Basics
ISBN# 0-9684266-0-3
1. Stretching exercises. I. Bashford, Daphne, 1962-
   RA781.63.S77 1998   613.7'1   C98-910924-0

The Rejuvenators

The Rejuvenators is a company that provides access for health professionals from a variety of disciplines to interact and focus on preventive and therapeutic measures for the individual, group or organization.

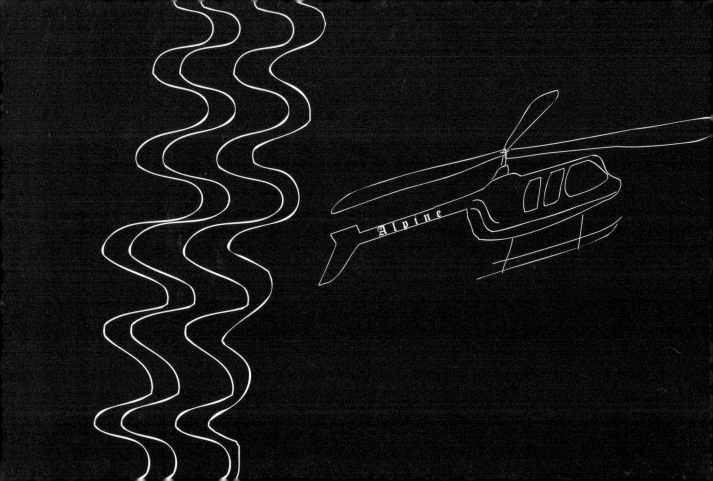

This book has been originally published for CMH (Canadian Mountain Holidays Heli Skiing and Heli Hiking) as a part of their ever-increasing safety and injury prevention program.

We thank them for being so open minded and hope it may encourage other organizations to move in the same direction. Proper stretching not only helps to relax the muscles and improve the body's range of motion, it also reduces general stress and tension. This allows for more fluid movement and responsive thought, as well as quicker reflex action. Safety, injury prevention and increased productivity are naturally promoted.

"Human beings often hesitate to make a beginning because they feel the objective cannot be achieved.

This attitude of mind is our greatest obstacle to progress."

M.K. Gandhi

For all the 'teachers' who give

us the inspiration and tools to maintain and rejuvenate ourselves.

We thank our diverse cross-section of clients who have requested such a book to help them help themselves.

v

Foreword

In my practice of Physical Medicine and Rehabilitation, I treat all kinds of musculoskeletal injuries. If there is a universal truth in medicine, it is that stretching is a necessary component of any treatment program for these injuries. Why not take the time to use this excellent stretching manual to start your injury prevention program. Look at the pictures, ask questions, think of it as insurance, so you can be active for longer.
Gregg Singer, M.D. • U.S.A.

Take yourself on a daily excursion into the world of stretching and flexibility. By following the suggestions in this amazing book you will improve the quality of your life – mind, body and soul. You will be able to perform at an optimum level. Treat yourself – stretch, breathe, be flexible. IT'S A WAY OF LIFE.
Shanne Leavitt, Former member of the Canadian National Alpine Ski Team, Coach and program director for Alberta Snowboarding Association and Professional T.V./Film stunt person • CANADA

Using the principles incorporated throughout this little gem of a manual will increase your appreciation and knowledge of your body. In turn, the pure joy of movement and the thrill of performance can only be enhanced. Indulge!
Shauna Zukiwsky, Movement Analyst/Personal Coach • CANADA

In this beautiful book everyone can find inspiration to learn about proper movement.
Peter Kraft, Occupational Therapist • SWEDEN

Doing heavy exercise without the addition of a well-rounded conditioning program is akin to driving a car that has not been properly maintained. Sooner or later they will both break down. The older the car, the more maintenance and tender loving care necessary.
Neil Ostrer, Money Manager, former Marathon Runner. A heli skier whose week of skiing was cut in half due to lower back problems • ENGLAND

Stress demands management. Ageing insists upon flexibility. "Stretch" enables the fulfillment of these realities.
Alan Hunter, Code Hunter Wittmann - Barristers & Solicitors • CANADA

Preface

It is difficult to pinpoint where the inspiration came from to create and produce this book. In part it has come from my insatiable desire to communicate my discoveries to a large and broad audience.

It has been my good fortune to invest the last ten years of my life into learning primarily about preventive and therapeutic health measures. I have practiced massage therapy for eight years and have spent many hours in yoga classes with world-renowned instructors. Having taken all this time to learn "hands on", I understand the struggle my clients have. Their area of expertise demands a professional focus of a different sort. Therefore, it is almost impossible to invest an equal amount of time and/or money to gain this invaluable knowledge about the body, which forms the foundation from which all else stems. The information in this book brings together, in a brief format, much of what my associates and I have learned over the years.

This is our gift to you – a concise manual to encourage the beginning of a simple yet comprehensive preventive health program. Proper stretching is one of the most fundamental things you can do for yourself to improve overall health. It is difficult to observe people spending hours of invaluable time stretching incorrectly. It gives us great pleasure to share our knowledge with you.

Joanne and Deanna are both experienced massage therapists who have been involved in fitness training for over ten years. Cynthia is a certified yoga instructor who specializes in its preventive and therapeutic benefits. She also contributes her knowledge gained from twenty years of dance training. Our expertise is similar yet varied. Most importantly our philosophy is the same: LIVE WHILE YOU LIVE!

Mobilize the shoulders, hips and pelvic girdle and the spine will naturally follow with ease. This is of utmost importance as all of our nerves pass through the spine.

Daphne Bashford

This book is a synthesis of knowledge gathered from years of study and work experience with thousands of people.

The basic stretch routine from years past has evolved dramatically. As with everything in today's world, it is important to update one's knowledge base. This is especially true when related to our own bodies, for if our health is compromised, everything we do will be affected.

The content of this book is basi
However, the attention to deta
provides for precision which i
necessary in a stretching program o
any level. *These concepts can and d
carry over to any movement we make
whether it be in sport, leisure o
work related situations*

VIII

" Do not kill the instinct of the body for the glory of the pose. Do not look at your body like a stranger , but adopt a friendly approach towards it. Watch it, listen to it, observe its needs, its requests, and even have fun. Play with it as children do, sometimes it becomes very alert and swift.

To be sensitive is to be alive."

Vanda Scaravelli, *Awakening The Spine*

● C A U T I O N

This program is not meant to replace advice given to you by health/medical professionals.

Please consult your physician if you
- are pregnant
- have had physical problems, surgery or have been inactive for a lengthy period
- feel unusual pain or discomfort while stretching.

ⓧ

C o n t e n t s

How to get the most out of this book

Comment profiter au maximum de ce livre

Tipps ober wie man den größten nutzen aus diesem buch erzielt

Come ottenere il massimo benefico da questo libro

Como aprovechar al maximo este libro

この本の最も効果的な使用方

1. The stretches in this book are organized into four routines. Doing just one out of the four routines can provide a suggested minimum amount of stretching to do each day.

- Les Ètirements dans ce livre s'organisent en quatre routines. Il vous suffira, dans bien des cas, de faire une seule routine parmi les quatre pour atteindre le niveau minimal d'Ètirements qu'il faut chaque jour.

- Die Dehnungen in diesem Buch sind in vier Übungen unterteilt. Jede Übung erfüllt die vorgeschlagene Mindestanzahl pro Tag für Dehnungen.

- Gli esercizi descritti sono organizzati in quattro diverse sequenze. L'esecuzione giornaliera di una sola delle sequenze puo` gia` rappresentate il numero minimo di esercizi di stretching consigliato.

- Los ejercicios de estiramiento que contiene este libro est·n organizados en cuatro rutinas. El ejecutar tan sölo una de las cuatro rutinas puede proporcionar el monto mÌnimo sugerido de estiramiento a realizarse todos los dÌas.

- この本に書かれた伸びの運動は四つの型にまとめられています。その型の一つを実行すれば、一日に
最低必要とみなされる伸びの運動量が得られるようになっています。

2. Aim to work through all four routines in one week. If you wish, do more than one routine in a day.
- Visez à faire les quatre routines en une semaine. Si vous voulez, vous pourriez faire plus d'une routine par jour.
- Man sollte versuchen möglichst alle vier Übungen wöchentlich auszuführen. Je nach Bedarf kann auch mehr als eine Übung an einem Tag gemacht werden.
- Cercate di eseguire tutte quattro le sequenze nel corso di una settimana. Se desiderate, eseguite piu` di una sequenza al giorno.
- Debe tener como objetivo el ejecutar las cuatro rutinas en el curso de una semana. Si lo desea, puede ejecutar m·s de una rutina al dìa.
- 一週間で四つの型の運動を全て実行する事を目標にしてください。ご希望の方は一日に一つ以上の型 の運動をしてください。

s	m	t	w	t	f	s
routine 1	routine 2	routine 3&4		routine 1&2		any routine

3. Integrate the stretch program into your daily routine.
- Intègrez le programme d'étirements dans votre routine quotidienne.
- Das Dehnungsprogramm sollte möglichst ein Bestandteil einer täglichen Routine werden.
- Integrate il programma di stretching con le vostre abitudini quotidiane.
- Integre el programa de ejercicios de estiramiento a su rutina diaria.
- 毎日の運動に伸びの運動を組み入れてください。

4. Represents the suggested minimum number of minutes to spend in the stretch sequence.
- Montre le nombre minimal de minutes que nous suggÈrons pour chaque Ètirement ou pour chaque groupe d'exercices.
  - Bezeichnet das Minimum der vorgeschlagenen Zeitdauer in Minuten für die Dehnung oder Serie von Übungen.
  - Rappresenta la minima quantita` di tempo consigliata per ogni esercizio o sequenza di esercizi.
  - Representa el n·mero mìnimo sugerido de minutos que debe de emplear en el ejercicio de estiramiento o la secuencia.
- は伸びやシークエンスに最低必要とみなされる、分単位の長さです。

5. Shows a deeper stretch. It tends to be advanced. Take your time.
  - Montre un étirement plus en profondeur et qui aura tendance à être plus avancé. Ne vous dépêchez pas.
  - Bezeichnet eine tiefergehende, kompliziertere Dehnung. Nehmen Sie sich Zeit.
  - Indica un esercizio eseguito in maggior profondita` e progressivamente piu` avanzato. Fate con comodo e seguite i vostri tempi.
  - Representa un ejercicio de estiramiento m·s intenso. Este ejercicio es a nivel avanzado. Tome su tiempo para hacerlo.
- は深い伸びの運動です。これは少し難しいかもしれないので、時間をかけて行ってください。

6. Shows a variation. It may be easier or simply different.
- Montre une variation qui peut être plus facile ou tout simplement un peu différent.
- Bezeichnet eine Variation. Sie kann leichter sein oder auch einfach anders.
- Indica un esercizio alternativo che puo` essere piu` facile o semplicemente diverso.
- Muestra una variante. Esta variante puede ser m·s f·cil o simplemente diferente.
- は少々変化を加えたものです。少し易しめか、或いは単に異なっているものです。

7. The body functions as an entire unit. When any movement is made, the whole body participates. Our detailed notes help you work with your body to its greatest benefit.
- Le corps fonctionne comme un tout. Quand vous faites un mouvement, tout le corps y participe. Les notes détaillées que nous fournissons vous aidera à donner un maximum de bénéfices à votre corps.
- Der Körper funktioniert als eine Einheit. Sobald eine Bewegung gemacht wird, wird der ganze Körper in Anspruch genommen. Unsere detaillierten Anweisungen helfen Ihnen mit Ihrem Körper am optimalsten umzugehen.
- Il nostro corpo funziona come una sola unita` ed e` coinvolto integralmente nell'esecuzione di ogni esercizio. Le nostre istruzioni dettagliate vi aiuteranno ad ottenere per il vostro organismo il massimo beneficio.
- El cuerpo funciona como una sola unidad. Cuando se ejecuta cualquier movimiento, todo el cuerpo participa. Nuestras anotaciones en detalle le ayudar·n a trabajar en conjunto con su cuerpo para que Èste se beneficie al m·ximo.
- 体の動きを総体的なユニットと考えてください。どのような動きも、全身が参加していなければなり ません。
  最大限の効果が得られるよう、この本の詳細をご参照ください。

8. Wear non-binding clothing. Stretch in your bare feet.
- Portez des vêtements amples et non-serrés.
- Tragen Sie lockere Kleidung und machen Sie alle Dehnübungen barfuß.
- Indossate capi comodi e non troppo stretti e rimanete a piedi nudi.
- Use ropa que permita libertad de movimiento. Estìrese con los pies descalzos.
- 体の動きに支障をきたさない服を着用してください。伸びの運動は、はだしでしてください。

9. Gather your supports (chair, blanket, strap, etc.) for each routine before starting.
- Rassemblez vos appuis (chaise, couverture, lanière, ...) pour chaque routine avant de commencer.
- Besorgen Sie sich alle Ihre Sachen vor dem Beginn jeder Übung (Stuhl, Decke, Gurt, usw.....) .
- Preparate in anticipo gli articoli necessari (sedia, coperta, cinghia, ecc.).
- Reuna todos los elementos de apoyo (silla, frazada, liga, etc.) para cada rutina antes de empezarla.
- それぞれの運動に必要な道具（椅子、毛布、ひも、ｅｔｃ．）は事前に用意しておいてください。

10. You should be able to comfortably hold each stretch for 20 seconds or more. If you feel pain, ease off. Do not bounce or overstretch. Your breathing should remain calm.
- Vous devriez être capable de tenir chaque étirement sans vous gêner pendant 20 secondes au moins. Si vous ressentez de la douleur, détendez-vous. Ne faites ni mouvements brusques ni mouvements excessifs.
- Sie sollten in der Lage sein jede Dehnung mindestens 20 Sekunden lang beizubehalten. Wenn es schmerzt, etwas nachgeben. Nicht überfedern oder überdehnen. Immer ruhig durchatmen.
- Dovreste poter mantenere ogni posizione di stretching 20 secondi o piu`. Se sentite male diminuite l'intensiata`. Evitate movimenti di scatto e allungamanti eccessivi. Respirate con calma.
- Debe ser capaz de mantener cada ejercicio de estiramiento con comodidad durante 20 segundos o m·s. Si siente dolor, deje de estirarse. No rebote ni se exceda en el estiramiento. Su respiración debe mantenerse calmada.
- 伸びの運動はそれぞれ、２０秒間又はそれ以上、そのままの姿勢を楽に保てるはずです。痛みを感じ
た場合はくつろいでください。はね返ったり、伸ばし過ぎたりしないようにしてください。呼吸は静
かに保ってください。

11. Never hold your breath. Coordinate your breathing with the stretch by inhaling when you lengthen, and exhaling when you relax deeper in the stretch.
- Ne retenez jamais votre souffle. Il faut coordoner votre respiration avec chaque étirement. Inspirez en vous allongeant puis expirez tout en vous détendant et en vous étirant plus en profondeur.
- Halten Sie nie den Atem an. Atem und Dehnung müssen übereinstimmen. Also gleichzeitig einatmen und dehnen; dann gegen Ende der Dehnung ausatmen und entspannen.
- Non trattenete il respiro ma coordinatelo col movimento. Inspirate mentre vi allungate ed espirate rilassandovi piu` profondamente nell'allungamento.
- Nunca retenga la respiraciòn. Coordine su respiraciòn con el estiramiento. Aspire y luego estìrese. Exhale y rel·jese m·s profundamente dentro del estiramiento.
- 呼吸を止めないでください。呼吸を伸びにコーディネートしてください。息を吸って伸びをし、息を
吐きながらリラックスし、更に深く伸びに入って行きます。

12. Do 2-3 shorter repetitions of your more challenging stretches. It will be more productive than doing 1 long stretch.
- Faites 2 ou 3 répétitions abrégées des étirements les plus exigeants ce qui sera plus rentable que de faire un seul étirement pendant plus longtemps.
- Bei den schwierigeren Dehnungen sind zwei oder drei wiederholte Dehnungen vorteilhafter, als eine lange Dehnung.
- Ripetete gli esercizi che trovate piu` difficili due o tre volte e per una durata minore; questo sara` piu` efficace di un solo e lungo esercizio di stretching.
- Repita 2 o 3 veces en forma breve los estiramientos más retadores para usted. Esto será más efectivo que el hacer 1 sólo estiramiento largo.
- 難しい伸びは、時間を短くし、２—３回繰り返してください。一回の長い伸びより効果的です。

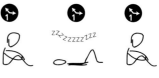

13. Always be sure to stretch each side of the body at least once. If you have a side that requires more attention, stretch it first and then come back to it again.
- Faites un étirement de chaque côté du corps au moins une fois. Si vous avez un côté qui a besoin d'attention plus que l'autre, commencez par faire des exercices de ce côté puis revenez-y un peu plus tard.
- Achten Sie darauf, dass jede Körperseite zumindest einmal gedehnt wird. Wenn eine Seite mehr Training benötigt, dehnen Sie diese zuerst und nochmals wieder am Schluss.
- Esercitate entrambi i lati del corpo almeno una volta. Se un lato richiede maggior attenzione dell'altro esercitatelo per primo e riesercitatelo successivamente.
- Asegúrese siempre de estirar por lo menos una vez cada lado del cuerpo. Si tiene un lado que requiere mayor atención, estire ese lado primero y luego regrese otra vez a ese mismo lado.
- 体の両側を最低一回ずつ伸ばしてください。もっと注目を要求されるサイドは、その片側から始め、再びそのサイドに戻り、もう一度伸ばしてください。

14. Listen to your body. Your flexibility will vary day by day and at different times during the day.
- Écoutez votre corps. Votre niveau de souplesse variera d'un jour à l'autre et à des moments différents de la journée.
- Hören Sie auf Ihren Körper. Ihre Flexibilität hängt von der Tageszeit ab und ändert sich täglich.
- Prestate attenzione al vostro corpo; il nostro livello di flessibilita` varia da un giorno all'altro e da un'ora all'altra.
- Preste atención a su cuerpo. Su flexibilidad variará de día y en día y en distintos momentos durante el día.
- 自分の体に充分注意を払ってみてください。柔軟性は、日毎に、或いは一日の内でも時間により異なります。

15. **Stretches can be done throughout the day. Take the book with you.**
* Les étirements peuvent se faire tout au long de la journée. Amenez ce livre avec vous.
* Dehnübungen können zu jeder Tageszeit gemacht werden. Nehmen Sie das Buch mit.
* Portate con voi questo libro; potete fare stretching in qualsiasi ora del giorno.
* Los estiramientos pueden ejecutarse a travÈs del dÌa. Lleve el libro consigo.
* 伸びの運動は一日を通していつでも行えます。本をいつも持っているようにしましょう。

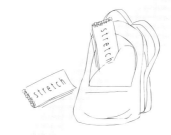

16. **We are 'doing' all day. Stretching is about 'undoing'.**
* Nous sommes en train de 'faire' chaque jour. Il s'agit, en faisant des étirements, se 'se remettre'.
* Wir sind den ganzen Tag angespannt. Dehnungsübungen dienen zum Entspannen.
* Ci 'carichiamo' tutto il giorno; con lo stretching ci 'scarichiamo'.
* Estamos "haciendo" todo el dÌa. Los ejercicios de estiramiento nos permiten "deshacer".
* 体は一日中使用されています。伸びの運動はその使用をほぐすものです。

Alignment

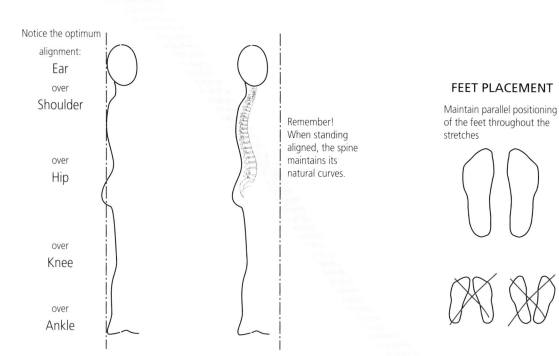

Notice the optimum alignment:

Ear
over
Shoulder

over
Hip

over
Knee

over
Ankle

Remember!
When standing aligned, the spine maintains its natural curves.

FEET PLACEMENT

Maintain parallel positioning of the feet throughout the stretches

Visualization

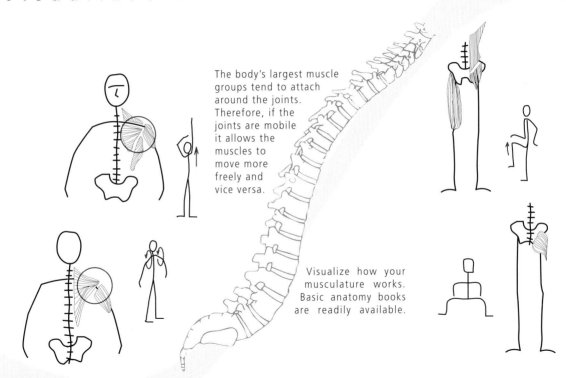

The body's largest muscle groups tend to attach around the joints. Therefore, if the joints are mobile it allows the muscles to move more freely and vice versa.

Visualize how your musculature works. Basic anatomy books are readily available.

Suggested Warmups

Always warmup before starting your routine.

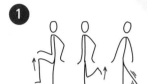

1 (A) Slowly bring knee up to waist height. Alternate legs.
(B) Bring leg behind. Alternate legs.
(C) Gently shake out legs from hip joint. Alternate legs.

Repeat 10 times on each leg. A, B, and C.

2 Bend knee up to hip height. Do outward rotating circles from hip joint. Alternate legs. Repeat 10 times each leg.

3 Lift straight leg out to the side. Alternate legs, repeat 3 times.

4 Twist upper body from side to side. Movement initiated from shoulders. Keep legs and hips stationary. Repeat 10 times to each side.

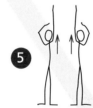

5 Hands up to head height. Gently reach upwards one arm at a time. Alternate arms. Repeat 6 times each arm.

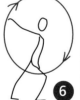

6 Slowly circle arms, one at a time. Opposite leg forward in a semi-lunge position. Circle forwards 4 times, then backwards 4 times. Lengthen out of shoulder joint.

7 Shoulder Shrugs: Lift both shoulders up to ear height, then let them relax down. Repeat approximately 8 times.

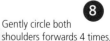

8 Gently circle both shoulders forwards 4 times, then backwards 4 times.

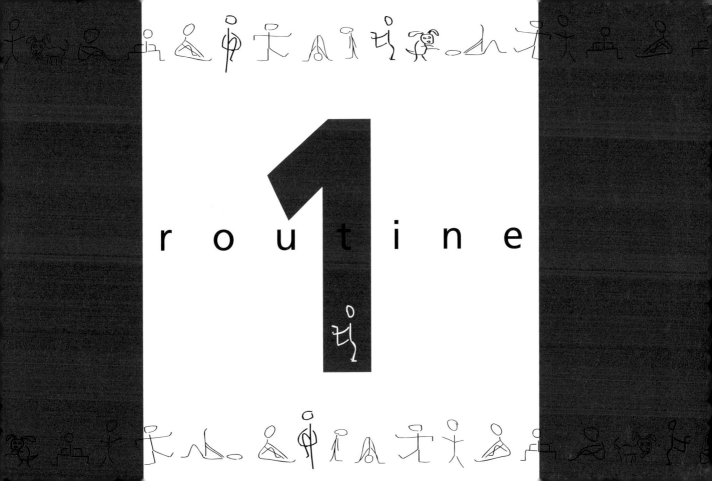

routine

1

Foot Stretch

 One minute - Do each side twice

DO NOT drop ankle out to the side

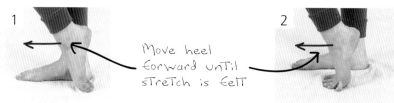

Move heel forward unTil sTreTch is felT

Stand straight to maintain length in body

Apply gentle pressure with toes pointing back

Apply gentle pressure with toes pointing forward

Ankle Stretch

 One minute - Do each side twice

- Shift most of your weight to standing leg
- Stabilize toes
- Draw a complete circle with ankle

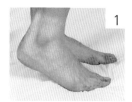 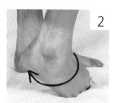 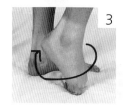 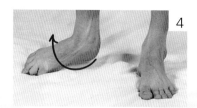

- Align and lengthen spine
- Straighten legs
- Stabilize toes

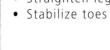

Ball of foot on book for support

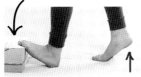

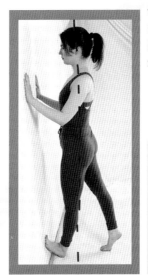

Back heel lifts while entire body shifts forward

Variation
Use wall for balance and support

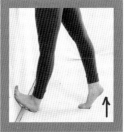

Hip and Ankle Rotation

 One minute - Rotate each direction twice

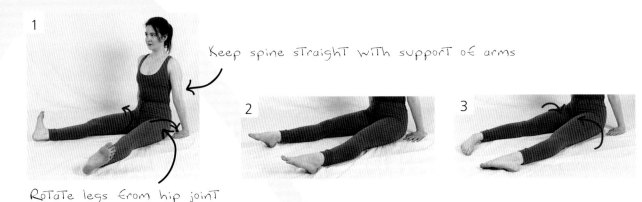

Keep spine straight with support of arms

Rotate legs from hip joint

Toes follow in a circular motion

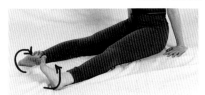 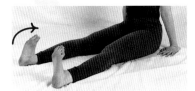

360°

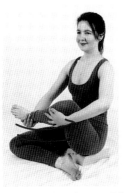

DO NOT round spine

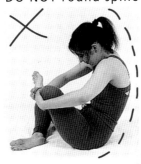

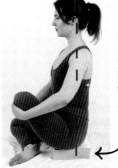

MainTain sTraighT spine wiTh use of supporT

- Rock leg from side to side
- Keep torso still

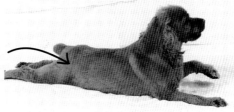

Wow, look aT These hips?

Inner Thigh Stretch Three minutes

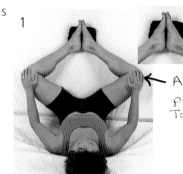

- Keep feet together
- Use padding for comfort

1

Apply genTle pressure To Thighs

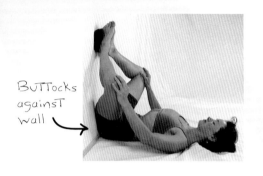

BuTTocks againsT wall

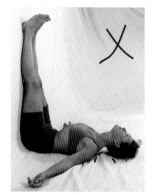

Keep buTTocks againsT wall if legs are comforTably sTraighT

Turn palms upward

Use head supporT

2

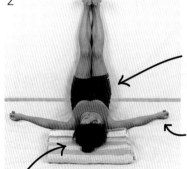

3

Slowly open legs

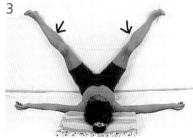

DO NOT
- overarch neck
- allow forehead to drop below level of chin

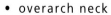

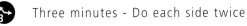

1

Use head support

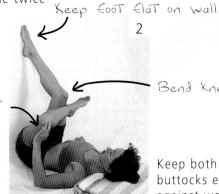

Keep foot flat on wall

2

Bend knee slightly

Apply gentle pressure to knee

Keep both buttocks evenly against wall

Variation
Easier version if needed

Knee closer to chest

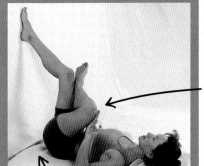

Buttocks away from wall

BREATHE!

Bring foot further down wall

3

Maintain gentle pressure on knee

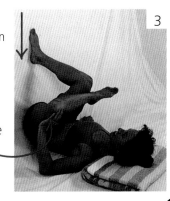

1 Extend heels away from body
Move toes toward body

With control, slowly lower legs

2

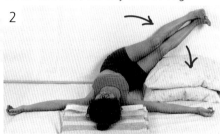

Direct Top buttock Toward wall. Don't let it fall forward.

3

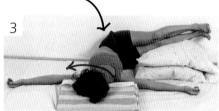

Throughout sequence keep
- feet flexed
- ankles together
- knees together
- shoulders pressed to floor
- buttocks against wall

Complete twist by turning head away from legs

BREATHE!

4

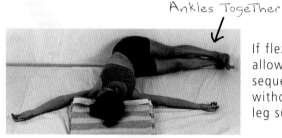

Ankles Together

If flexibility allows do sequence without leg support

Back difficulties? Bend legs to move between positions.

1

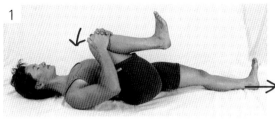

Extend through heel
to keep leg straight

- Bring knee toward chest
- Keep shoulders relaxed

2

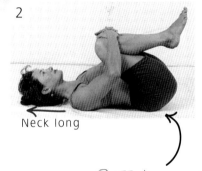

Neck long

BuTTocks remain
on floor

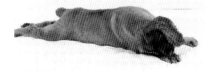

Ahhhh?

Notes

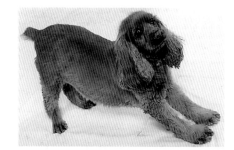

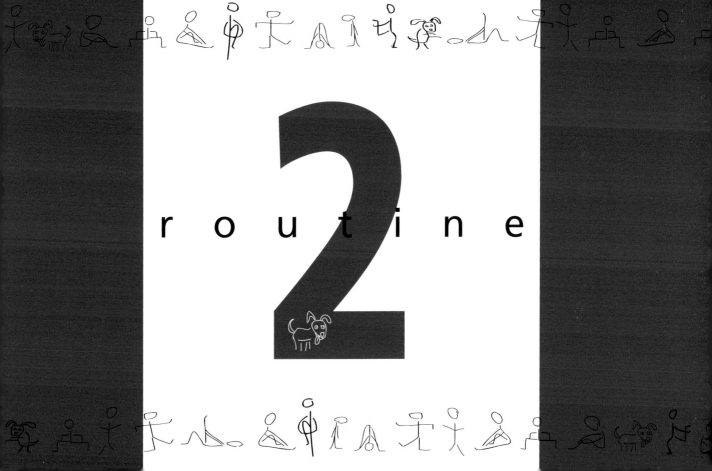

routine

2

Forward Bend

STAGE ONE One minute

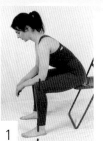

1

Sit on edge of chair with knees over ankles

Feel length in low back

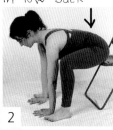

2

Keep entire spine straight

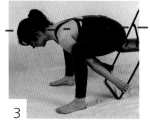

3

STAGE TWO One minute

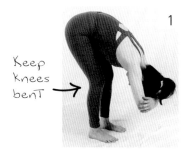

1

Keep knees bent

Relax upper body

BREATHE!

Straighten legs if flexibility allows

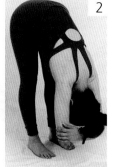

2

Lengthen spine with head and neck relaxed

STAGE THREE One minute

Press hands into wall
and extend out through
tailbone

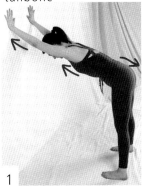

1

Move shoulders away
from ears and spine

- Move hands lower down wall
- Wrists do not fall below level
  of tailbone

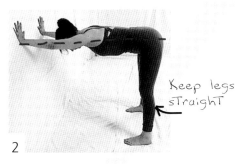

Keep legs
straight

2

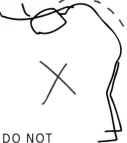

DO NOT
- drop head
- round back
- bend knees

DO NOT
- raise head
- overarch back
- hyperextend knees

 Move through the stages slowly. Use your breath to find more length
and ease in the body. Inhale and lengthen. Exhale and relax deeper
into the stretch

Forward Bend

STAGE FOUR One minute

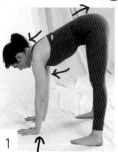

Spine and front of torso long

1

Wrists below shoulders

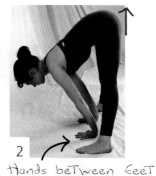

2

Hands between feet

- Tailbone moves upward
- Legs straight

Variation
Feet together

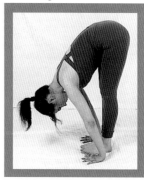

STAGE FIVE One minute

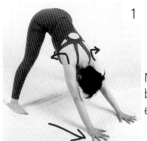

1

Move shoulder blades away from ears and spine

Walk hands away from feet

Relax head and neck downward

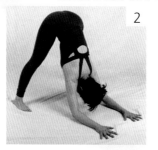

2

Rest elbows on floor if flexibility allows

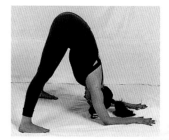

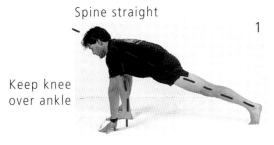

Spine straight

1

Keep knee
over ankle

BREATHE!

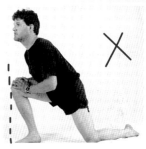

- Extend heel back to straighten leg
- Extend out of hip joint
- Let hips move toward floor

DO NOT move knee
beyond toes

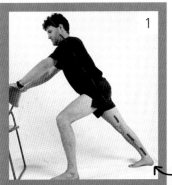

1

Easier Variation
Use chair for support

Create a straight
line with back leg
and spine

Heel on floor

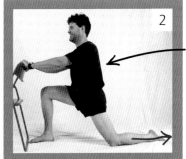

2

Keep
Torso
Upright

Move leg back to deepen stretch

Thigh Stretch

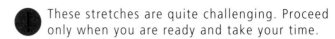 These stretches are quite challenging. Proceed only when you are ready and take your time.

WITH STRAP Two minutes - Do each side twice

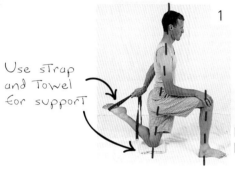

Use strap and Towel for support

1

Keep front knee over ankle

Extend arm overhead to open the shoulder

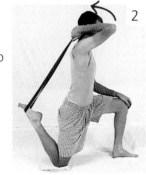

2 Move elbow up and back if flexibility allows

AT WALL Two minutes - Do each side twice

Keep lower leg against the wall

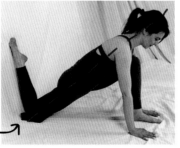

Use Towel for support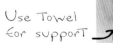

Create straight line with upper leg and spine

BREATHE!

While hips sink toward floor, lengthen spine upward

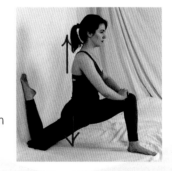

Torso shifts
toward bent leg

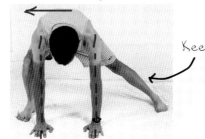

Keep leg sTraighT

Keep
• spine straight
• shoulders over wrists

To deepen stretch
• widen distance between feet
• increase bend in leg

Easier Variation
Use chair

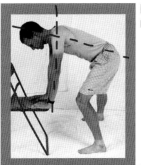

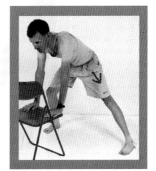

Extend out of
hip joint

Hamstring Stretch

 Two minutes - Do each side twice

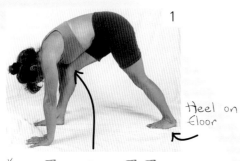

1

Heel on floor

Keep Torso in conTacT WiTh benT leg

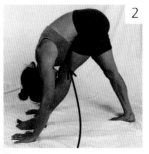

2

Keep Torso in conTacT WiTh sTraighTened leg

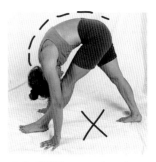

DO NOT round spine

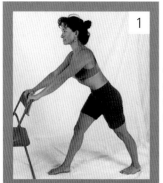

1

Variation
Use chair
for support

- Lengthen spine and arms
- Bend at hips
- Keep legs straight
- Keep back heel on floor

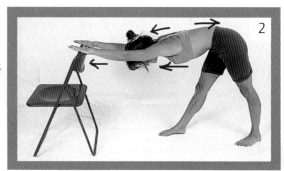

2

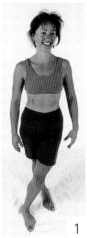

Bend both legs
slightly

1

Create a "C" curve

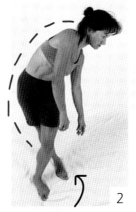

2

Weight primarily
on back leg

Extend torso
upward and over

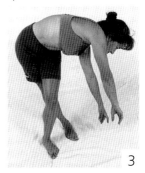

3

STAGE ONE Two minutes - Do each side twice

Move bent leg to opposite side of body

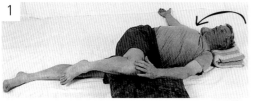

Keep shoulder on floor

Use support if knee does not reach floor

STAGE TWO Two minutes - Do each side twice

Keep shoulder on floor

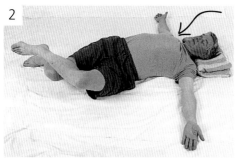

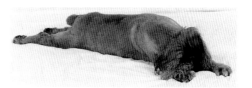

Zzzzzzz...

- Cross calf over opposite knee
- Allow knees to move toward floor

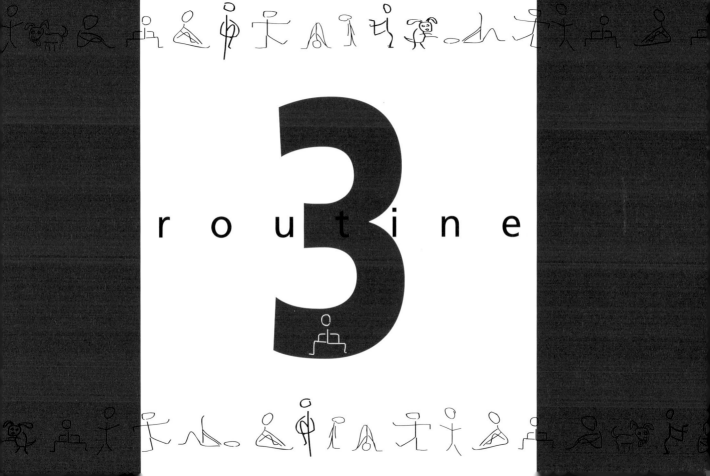

routine

3

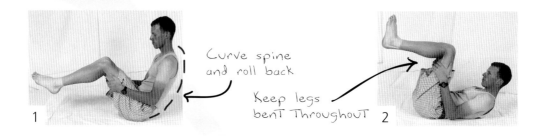

Curve spine and roll back

Keep legs bent throughout

1

2

Massage spine with movement

HAVE FUN AND BREATHE!

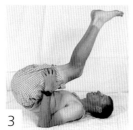

Roll through spine one vertebra at a time

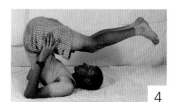

3

4

Come down and repeat

Keep upper back and shoulder blades on floor to protect neck.

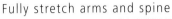
Fully stretch arms and spine

1

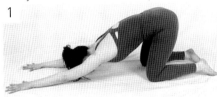

Move shoulders away from ears and spine

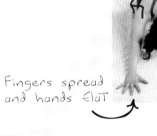

Fingers spread and hands flat

ELONGATE!

2

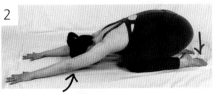

Move buttocks toward heels while maintaining length in upper body

Forehead rests on floor or a support

Knee to chest

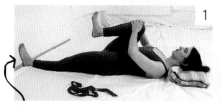

1

Press foot into wall to straighten leg

Place strap on ball of foot and extend heel away

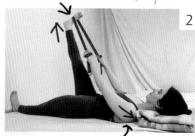

2

Shoulder relaxed on floor

BREATHE AND MOVE SLOWLY!

Arms and legs straight

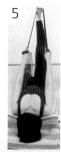

Use head support

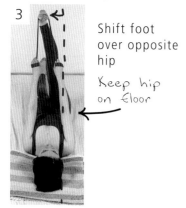

3

Shift foot over opposite hip

Keep hip on floor

Move hip away from lower ribs

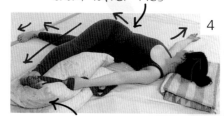

4

- Keep both shoulders on floor
- Turn head to opposite direction of leg

Use support under leg

5

Return to centre

Slowly extend leg outward

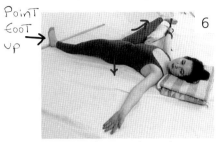

Point Foot Up →

6

Hip remains anchored to floor

Create straight line with torso and leg

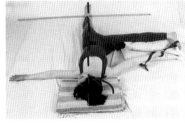

Turn head away from leg

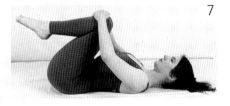

7

After completing both sides
- knees to chest
- relax and breathe

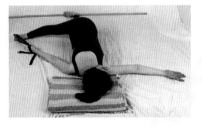

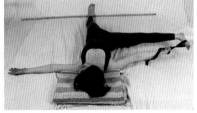

- If flexibility allows no support under leg
- Both shoulders remain relaxed on floor

34

Cat Stretch

Two minutes - Repeat sequence several times

Mid-spine arches upward with exhalation

Rediscover The spine!

Elongate spine

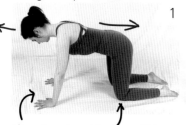

1

Hands shoulder-width apart and knees hip-width apart

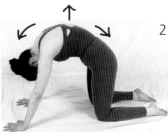

2

Relax head and tailbone down

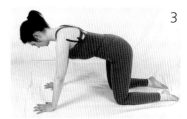

3

Shoulders move away from ears

Look at floor a few feet ahead

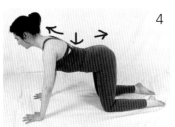

4

Head and tailbone tilt up

Mid-spine gently arches downward with inhalation

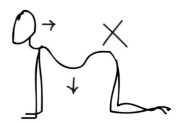

DO NOT overarch
• neck
• low back

Create maximum length in the spine throughout sequence.

Backbend

STAGE ONE   One minute - Repeat sequence several times

Keep body long with elbows and hands anchored throughout sequence

Move head up and away to begin back arch

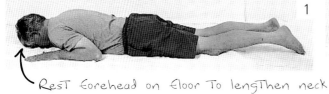

1

2

Rest forehead on floor to lengthen neck

Press forearms on floor to slowly raise upper body

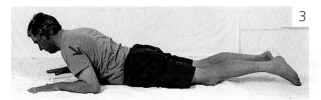

3

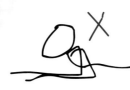

X

DO NOT
• lift and tilt head back
• move shoulders toward ears

• Look at floor
• Move shoulders toward hips

Return to floor by slowly moving vertebra by vertebra

 Keep neck and low back long.

36

STAGE TWO One minute - Repeat sequence several times

Keep elbows close to torso throughout sequence

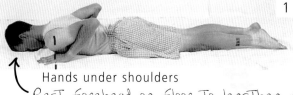

1

Hands under shoulders

ResT forehead on floor To lengThen neck

2

Move head up and away

Keep neck and low back long

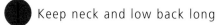

Press hands on floor to slowly raise upper body

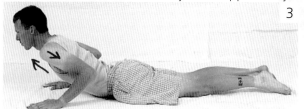

3

• Move shoulders toward hips
• Extend chest up and away

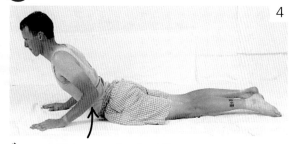

4

Arms can remain benT

Reverse movement to return to floor

Two minutes - Do each side twice

Twist toward wall

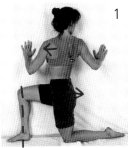

1

Move shoulders
and hips in
opposite
directions

Knee over ankle

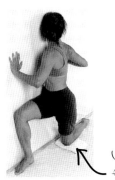

Use Towel
for Knee support

Arms wide

2

Keep shoulders level and pressurize hands to increase twist

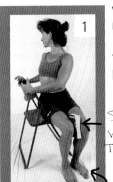

1

Variation
Use chair

Twist toward
back of chair

Squeeze book
with knees
to anchor hips

Feet flat on floor

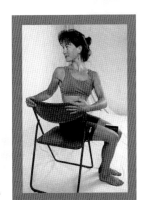

Gently turn head to complete twists

Bring knees
toward chest

Relax!

Notes

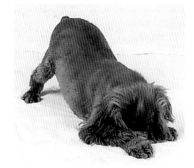

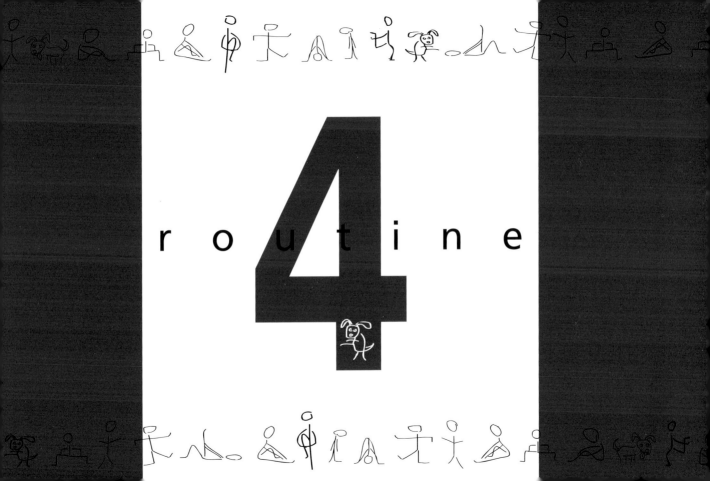

routine 4

🏃 6

Six minutes - Complete several rotations with arm and change sides

Throughout sequence
- extend in all directions
- press foot into wall
- keep bent knee resting on support
- move upper hip toward wall
- keep arms straight

270°

Use pillow and blanket for support

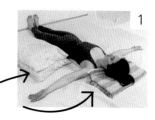

1

Place foot on knee

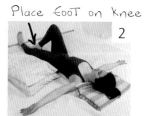

2

Toes point to side →

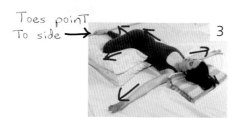

3

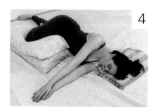

4

MOVE VERY SLOWLY AND EXTEND!

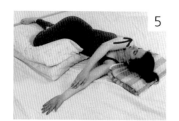

5

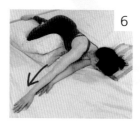

6

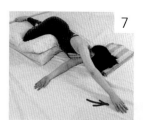

7

Repeat several times

Palm faces floor

Pause and release tight spots using the breath!

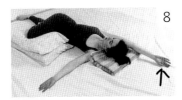 8

Palm Turns upward

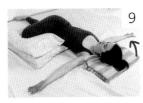 9

CREATE LENGTH!

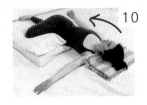 10

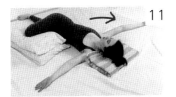 11

Now move in opposite direction

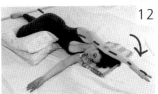 12

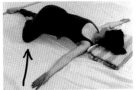

Remove leg support
if flexibility allows

Knee remains on floor

13

DO NOT force the stretch.
The moving hand and
shoulders DO NOT have to
touch the floor.

One minute
Do each side twice

Straighten arm

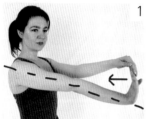

1

Apply gentle pressure
to fingers

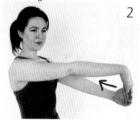

2

Standing Stretch

 Two minutes - Do each side twice

Create maximum length in The body

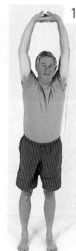

1

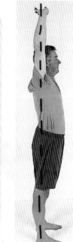

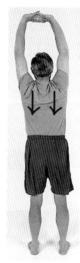

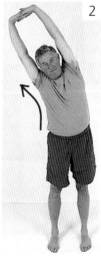

2

Maintain
length
on bent
side

- Feet under hips
- Interlace fingers
- Palms parallel
  to ceiling

- Arms straight
- Move shoulder
  blades toward
  hips

- Extend palms to ceiling
- Extend upward and
  to the side

Three minutes - Do each side twice

1

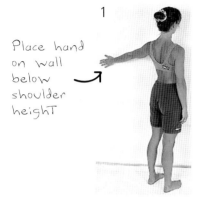

Place hand on wall below shoulder height

2

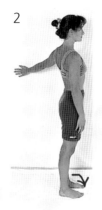

Stabilize hand and turn body away from wall

Keep shoulders level

Stand straight

3

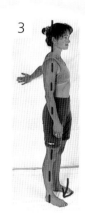

Continue turning away from wall to deepen stretch

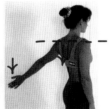

Move hand down wall if needed

Move shoulders downward

Keep low back long

HALF Two minutes - Do each side twice

Keep elbow close To head

Move hand down upper back

1

2

3

Move hand up spine

BREATHE!

FULL Two minutes - Do each side twice

Stand straight!

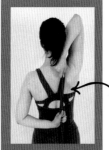

Variation
Use strap for support

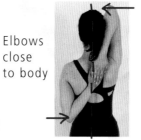

Elbows close to body

Hands meet

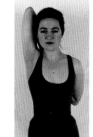

DO NOT drop head forward or arch low back

Two minutes - Do each side twice

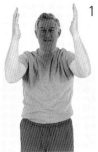

1

Elbows at shoulder height

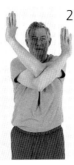

2

Cross one arm over the other

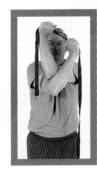

Variation
With strap

Move hands together

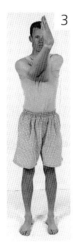

3

Bring palms together if flexibility allows

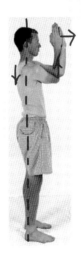

Move
- shoulders down
- elbows up
- hands away from face

STAND STRAIGHT AND BREATHE!

Neck Stretch

 Two minutes - Do each side twice

Press head into hand to deepen stretch

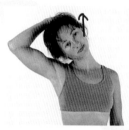

- Extend ear upward
- Move shoulder blades downward

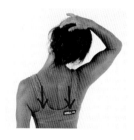

 Maintain length. **DO NOT strain neck!**

Head Rotation

 Two minutes - Repeat several times

180°

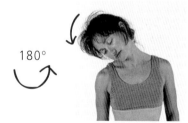 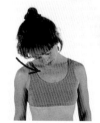 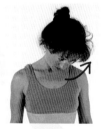 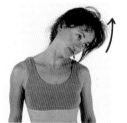

Slowly create semi-circles with head

 DO NOT extend head back

Recommended Reading

Acu-Yoga, Michael Reed Gach with Carolyn Marco
Awakening The Spine, Vanda Scaravelli
Back Care Basics, Mary Pullig Schatz, M.D.
Yoga The Iyengar Way, Silva, Mira and Shyam Mehta

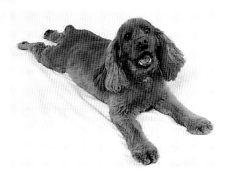

Anatomical Index

Our stretches tend to benefit the entire body, however, the following reference provides information for specific focus.

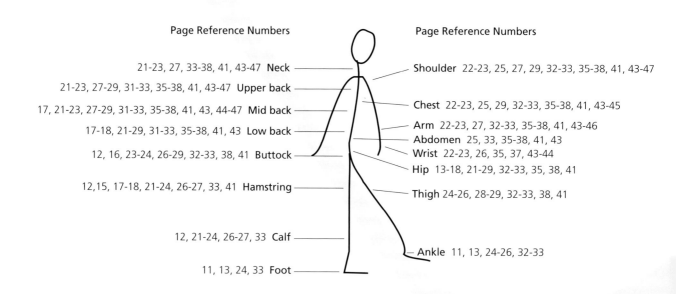

Page Reference Numbers

21-23, 27, 33-38, 41, 43-47 **Neck**

21-23, 27-29, 31-33, 35-38, 41, 43-47 **Upper back**

17, 21-23, 27-29, 31-33, 35-38, 41, 43, 44-47 **Mid back**

17-18, 21-29, 31-33, 35-38, 41, 43 **Low back**

12, 16, 23-24, 26-29, 32-33, 38, 41 **Buttock**

12,15, 17-18, 21-24, 26-27, 33, 41 **Hamstring**

12, 21-24, 26-27, 33 **Calf**

11, 13, 24, 33 **Foot**

Page Reference Numbers

Shoulder 22-23, 25, 27, 29, 32-33, 35-38, 41, 43-47

Chest 22-23, 25, 29, 32-33, 35-38, 41, 43-45

Arm 22-23, 27, 32-33, 35-38, 41, 43-46

Abdomen 25, 33, 35-38, 41, 43

Wrist 22-23, 26, 35, 37, 43-44

Hip 13-18, 21-29, 32-33, 35, 38, 41

Thigh 24-26, 28-29, 32-33, 38, 41

Ankle 11, 13, 24-26, 32-33

A c k n o w l e d g e m e n t s

Thank goodness for and Thank you To good friends, family, and dogs. Without Their never-ending support, advice and love This book would not exist.

An extra special Thanks To Gregg, Shane, Shauna, Peter, Neil, and Alan who offered Their support, advice, honest critiques, and endorsements in The foreword.

Special Thanks To: Kallen Graphics and Corinne Cowell Design for saving The day; our private bankers for not making institution-like decisions; David Moore for his number crunching education; David McAmmond for providing our foundation; Cynthia Palahniuk for being so nitpicky and for working with me until sunrise on many occasions; Deanna Empey and Joanne Boston for helping To ignite and maintain The fire; Sandy and Miles Prodan for Too many Things To write down; Shane Leavitt and Lisa Downing for Their humour and inspiration; Sean Beaumont for enduring my constant barrage of questions about everything and for helping out with The design; Romana Prokopiw for owning such a great bookstore (Books and Books, Calgary, Alberta) whose beautiful books provided much inspiration; Roger Laing for putting up with us; Alan and Ginney Hunter for being The way They are; Nick Kirton for never giving up on me; and Mumma, Papa, and Pisco for always being There. Finally I Thank Gummy for, no matter what, believing in me — wherever you are now... Salud?

The publisher and authors wish to thank HarperCollins publishers for allowing use of the Vanda Scaravelli quote, from "*Awakening the Spine*" 1991 pg. 38.

Design Concept by	Daphne Bashford
Printed in Canada by	Kallen Graphics Ltd.
Graphic Design by	Corinne Cowell Design Inc.
Translation by	Action Communications International Calgary
Text Editing by	Romana Prokopiw and Cynthia Palahniuk
Stretch Editing by	Cynthia Palahniuk and David McAmmond
Photography by	Roger Laing
Models:	Alan Hunter, Roger Laing, Jake Gotta, Cynthia Palahniuk, Deanna Empey and Pisco

Muchas Gracias,
Daphne Bashford

If your organization would like to order this book or
have us develop one to better suit your needs,
please contact us. Workshops and seminars can also
be arranged.

Pisco

Press

Pisco Press
Box 130
100, 1039 - 17 Avenue S.W.
Calgary, Alberta, CANADA
T2T 0B2

Fax: (403) 244-2431

E-mail: pisco@telusplanet.net

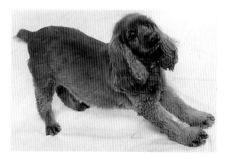